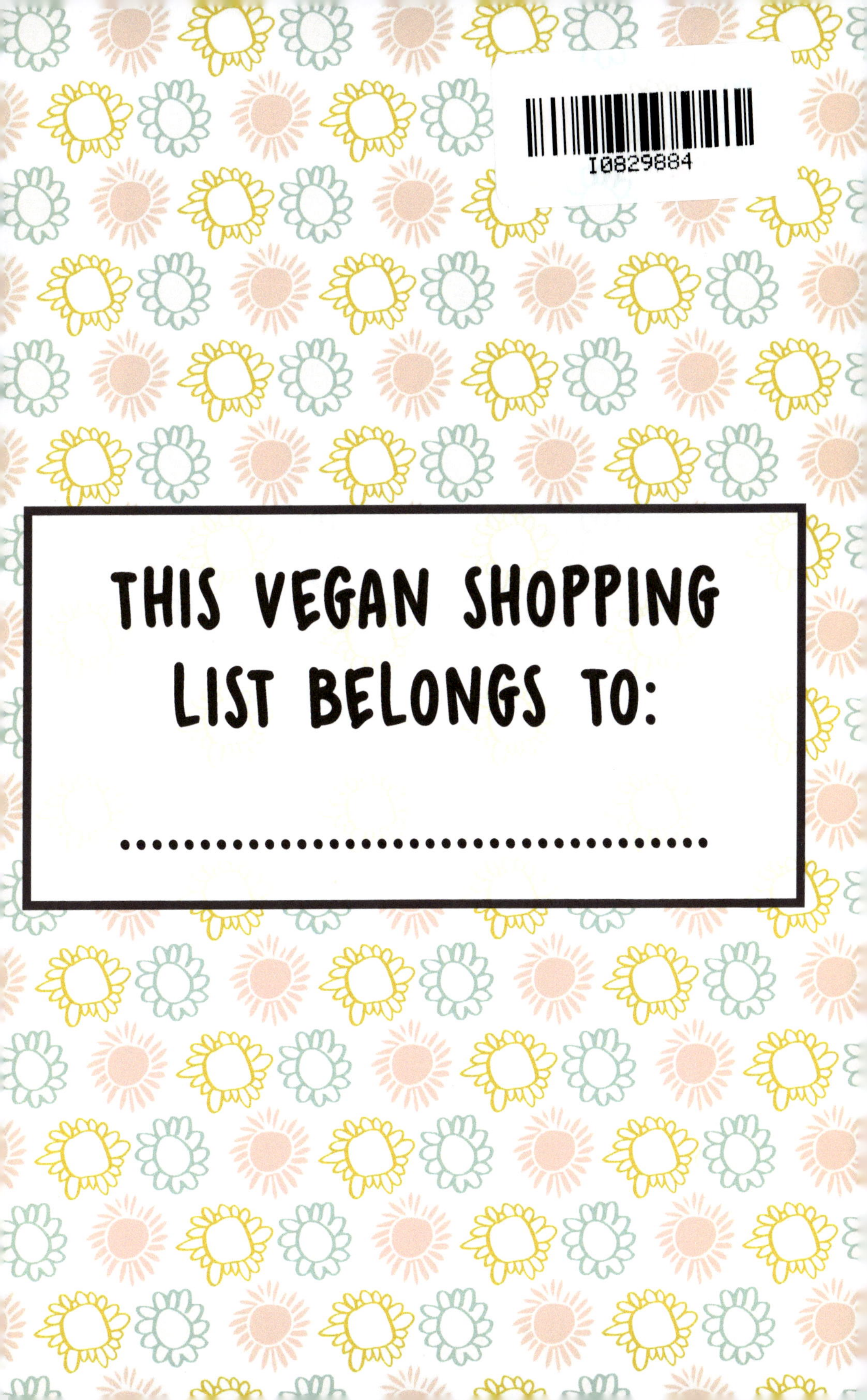
THIS VEGAN SHOPPING
LIST BELONGS TO:

....

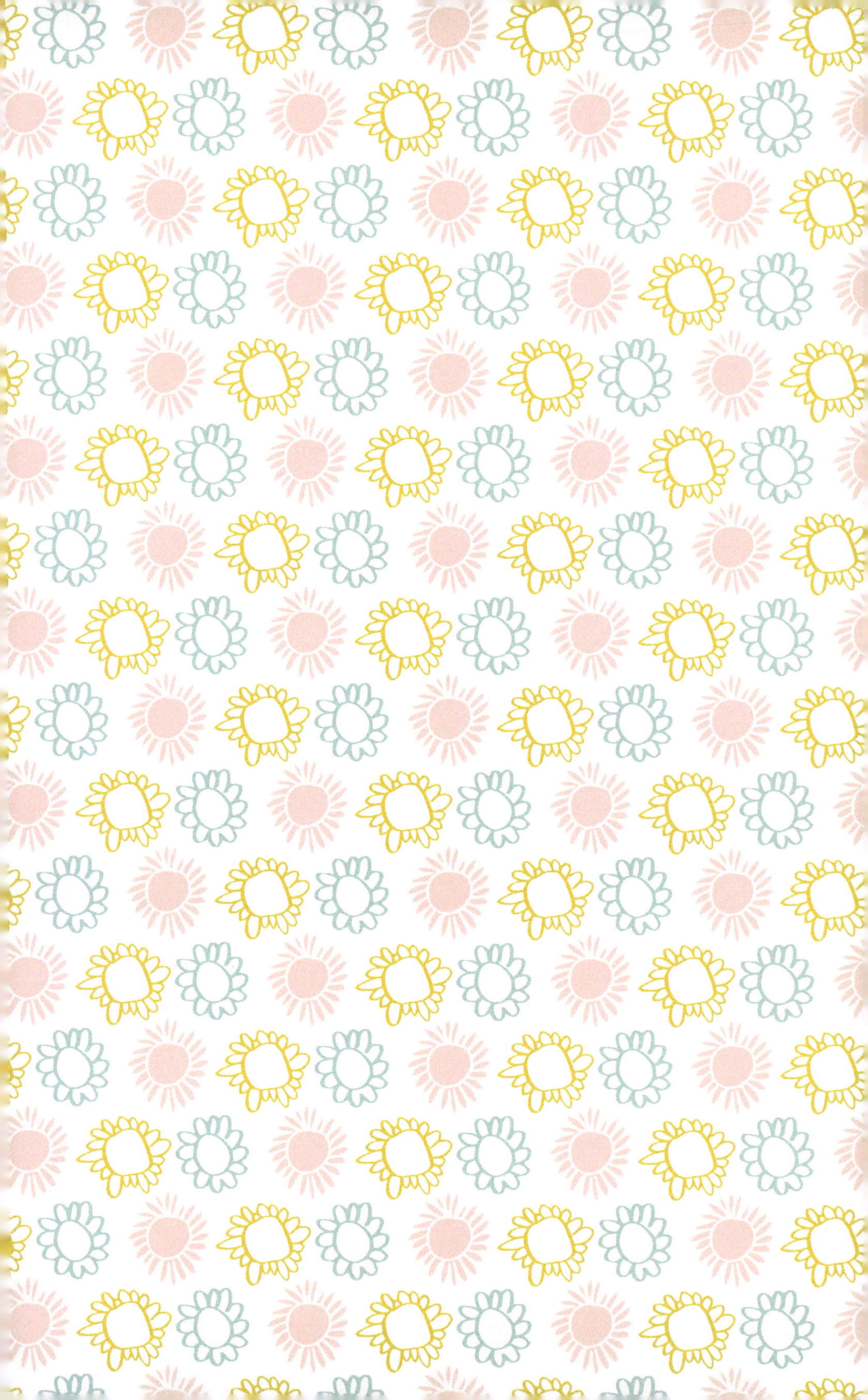

MY VEGAN SHOPPING LIST

MY VEGAN SHOPPING LIST

MY VEGAN SHOPPING LIST

MY VEGAN SHOPPING LIST

MY VEGAN SHOPPING LIST

MY VEGAN SHOPPING LIST

MY VEGAN SHOPPING LIST

MY VEGAN SHOPPING LIST

MY VEGAN SHOPPING LIST

MY VEGAN SHOPPING LIST

MY VEGAN SHOPPING LIST

MY VEGAN SHOPPING LIST

MY VEGAN SHOPPING LIST

MY VEGAN SHOPPING LIST

MY VEGAN SHOPPING LIST

MY VEGAN SHOPPING LIST

MY VEGAN SHOPPING LIST

MY VEGAN SHOPPING LIST

MY VEGAN SHOPPING LIST

MY VEGAN SHOPPING LIST

MY VEGAN SHOPPING LIST

MY VEGAN SHOPPING LIST

MY VEGAN SHOPPING LIST

MY VEGAN SHOPPING LIST

MY VEGAN SHOPPING LIST

MY VEGAN SHOPPING LIST

MY VEGAN SHOPPING LIST

MY VEGAN SHOPPING LIST

MY VEGAN SHOPPING LIST

MY VEGAN SHOPPING LIST

MY VEGAN SHOPPING LIST

MY VEGAN SHOPPING LIST

MY VEGAN SHOPPING LIST

MY VEGAN SHOPPING LIST

MY VEGAN SHOPPING LIST

MY VEGAN SHOPPING LIST

MY VEGAN SHOPPING LIST

MY VEGAN SHOPPING LIST